3x - 11.5 Wide

3x - 11.5 Wide

One Woman's Journey

<u>Dedication</u>

I dedicate this experience to

Fat Secret™

Fat Secret™ is one of my most valuable tools, so vital to my weight loss and the continuing restoration of my well being.

The Journey Begins

I started out as a long distance runner at the age of 16.

I would run the hills close to my home; running 5 miles or more each day.

I was 5'9' and weighed a lean, muscular 160 pounds.

I continued running until I became very Ill in my 30's and 40's.

I was struck with Bipolar illness and Rheumatoid Arthritis at the same time.

To this day, I still need to take medications for both illnesses.

I ballooned up to 282 pounds and had what looked like a pregnant belly due to my Bipolar medications.

This weight gain was also due to inactivity brought on by the Rheumatoid Arthritis.

This is my story as I transformed from a lean, beautiful body to become a size 3x clothes size and a size 11.5 wide shoes and my continuing road to recovery.

Table of Contents

Being Bipolar (1)

Being Bipolar, until treatment is achieved, is like being on a Ferris wheel without the controls.

You go up, you go down, non-stop.

I always knew something was wrong with me when I was younger when my moods vacillated from way up to way down.

The extremes continued into my thirties and culminated in my forties.

I was diagnosed when I ended up in a mental hospital in my thirties and spent two weeks there.

I went through a slew of testing and drugs until my diagnosis emerged – Bipolar I.

Bipolar I is the severest form of Bipolar illness.

Normally with Bipolar I disorder there is an episode of psychosis.

My psychosis manifested in my early thirties when I thought I was in hell.

I literally couldn't distinguish if I was on earth or in hell.

It was an out of this world experience.

As a result, this turned out to be my first of four mental hospital stays.

I was lucky to find a fantastic psychiatrist the fourth time around and am overjoyed that I am completely stabilized now.

Having Rheumatoid Arthritis (2)

I was broad-sided with Rheumatoid Arthritis (RA) in my forties.

RA hit me like a semi-truck.

My mom had some Osteo Arthritis, which according to my experience is not as severe as having RA.

My sisters never manifested signs of the illness.

I suffered stoically through RA, not having anyone that could relate to my illness in my family. No one had experienced it.

At its worst it felt like my legs were on fire; not being able to move without extreme pain. At its best, there is no pain, just deformities of the hands and feet.

Deformities (3)

My feet and hands are deformed.

I experienced some deformity in my feet from the RA. It made my feet spread out.

The toes go left or right away from the big toe.

Thus, the 11.5 size wide.

As I've lost some weight, my feet are less swollen.

I am a size 11 now. Luckily, my feet have shrunk width wise.

I guess my wide feet were partly to blame on my weight gain.

My hands are another story. I have had several unsuccessful surgeries to correct the Ulnar drift I now have.

Orencia (4)

Thank God for modern medicine.

I tried several immunosuppressant drugs without success until I tried Orencia, which is what I take as a monthly infusion.

It is my miracle. My saving grace.

And as a result of the Orencia, I am basically pain free and fully mobile.

With the RA under control, I am freed up to work on my weight.

What it's Like Being Overweight (5)

I feel very ugly being overweight.

Guys don't look at me.

If they do, they look through me or avert their stare when I catch them staring at my belly.

Not a stare of admiration, but a stare of repulsion.

This is foreign to me.

Throughout my life I was always complimented on my looks.

I was a cheerleader and I enjoyed all that came with this popularity.

As a runner I always had a shapely figure; athletic, but not manly.

Being overweight, I remember going to Disneyland. I had to get one of those electric carts because I couldn't walk very far without resting.

I was surprised to learn that people didn't get out of the way unless they absolutely had to, leaving me to navigate through a sea of people.

I was someone to be avoided, not accommodated.

That felt really, really bad.

When I got off the electric cart, at least I was able to see people at eye level.

I felt less ostracized – less of the worst.

On the opposite extreme, my husband always makes me feel pretty.

My husband finds something each day to compliment me on – my face, weight loss (even if I just lose one pound), and the clothes that I buy.

Resources (6)

Fat Secret™

Fat Secret™, my husband and my family's encouragement are all responsible for my continuing weight loss.

Fat Secret™ is a website and a cell phone application.

It helps you see how many fat grams are in an item.

You can have fat, but you must keep it down to 65 grams of fat or below a day depending upon your desired weight loss.

Fat Secret™ also keeps a diary for you of what you eat and how it's broken down fat and calorie-wise.

Fat Secret™ tracks your weight and provides additional information on each food item.

I also limit my portions. I use a bowl instead of plates as a way to gauge my portions.

On weekends and when I'm going out to dinner I have my Fat Secret™ application on my phone to assist me in making wise food decisions.

Ultimately, Fat Secret™ is the tool that works the best for me.

Additional Resources (7)

Subway's™ 6 grams of fat or less sandwiches are very favorable as an addition to my weight loss regimen.

They help me one or two days during the week to continue my weight loss efforts while still feeling that I'm eating a substantial meal.

I feel healthy and satiated when I eat these sandwiches.

Along with Subway™, I sometimes add Progresso™ soups when I'm extra hungry.

The soups I choose are 5 grams or less of fat per serving. They have a variety of soups that fit this category.

Progresso™ soups are found in virtually every grocery store.

So you see I have a variety of food resources to keep me on track.

I also consume a variety of foods that are 0 grams of fat. Just check the label or use the Fat Secret™ application or its computer website.

Conclusion (8)

Having Bipolar Illness and/or Rheumatoid Arthritis is hard enough.

Complicate this situation with obesity.

What turns into a very difficult situation becomes intolerable.

What I have learned on my road to recovery from a life that some women experience on a daily basis, year after year, is that there is a way out.

By using these simple tools, I offer a genuine hope and a path out of the agony that is obesity.

Websites (9)

Subway™ www.Subway.com

Progresso™ www.Progresso.com

Fat Secret™ www.FatSecret.com

www.ALifeisShortPublication.com

<u>Notes</u>

Notes

<u>Notes</u>

Notes

Notes